Resilience and Purpose

Discovering Strength and Connection in Life's Cracks

Anne Mok

Finesse Literary Press Ltd.

Copyright © 2025 by Anne Mok.

All rights reserved.

No part of this book may be reproduced without written permission from the publisher or author, except as permitted by U.S. copyright law. The information provided is accurate to the best of the author's and publisher's knowledge but is not a substitute for professional advice. They make no warranties regarding its completeness or suitability and disclaim liability for any losses, including commercial or incidental damages. Consult a professional for specific guidance.

First edition 2025 published by Finesse Literary Press Ltd.

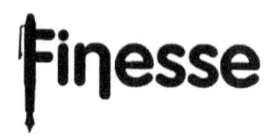

Finesse

Contents

Dedication — 1

Introduction — 3

The Breaking Point

1. Another Angel — 10
2. The Night That Redefined Us — 19
3. Blind Sighted: Seeing Beyond The Darkness — 28
4. Unrelenting Pain — 38

The Turning Point

5. Curiosity Leads to Change — 48
6. Shifting Perceptions of Blindness — 56
7. Breaking Barriers: Accessibility as a Path to Empowerment — 66

The Empowered Point

    8. Representation   76

    9. I Can Achieve That   90

    10. Becoming Each Other's Caregivers   101

Full Circle

    11. Advocating for Ourselves   112

    12. There is Light After Darkness   122

    13. A Call to Action   130

Conclusion   137

Acknowledgements   142

Endnotes   145

To my husband, Tony—your unwavering love, strength, and belief in me have been my anchor in every storm. Through every challenge, every triumph, and every quiet moment in between, you have been by my side, reminding me that love is both the foundation and the light that guides us forward.

To my children, Chenessa, Christopher, and Lauren—you are my greatest joy, my fiercest motivation, and my constant reminder that resilience is woven into the fabric of our family. You have each taught me the true meaning of courage, unconditional love, and the power of perseverance. Through my journey with vision loss and chronic illness, I have learned that the greatest lessons are often found in the spaces between the chapters—the quiet moments of struggle, the whispers of strength, and the choices we make when no one is watching.

I want you to always remember that even in the darkest moments, there is light waiting to be found. You are the authors of your own story, and your voice, your path, and your purpose are yours to shape. May you always walk forward with resilience, guided by love, and never forget that your story is still being written.

ANNE MOK

This book is as much yours as it is mine—because every step of this journey, every lesson, and every ounce of strength I have poured into these pages comes from the love we share.

Thank you for being my greatest inspiration.

Love, Anne

Introduction

The first time I used my white cane in public, my heart raced with fear and shame. The cane, a symbol of my visual impairment, represented my limitations, my loss of independence, and my fear. That was my perception at the time, and I was convinced that everyone saw me the same way. The world suddenly felt smaller, and I questioned my ability to navigate it with confidence. It would be months before that perception shifted—all because of a single message.

A young girl from halfway across the globe wrote to me, expressing how seeing someone who looked like her—a blind Asian woman—using a white cane had given her the courage to embrace her own story. From that day on, I saw my cane—and myself—in a new light. In her words, I found clarity and purpose. The girl's message reminded me that the journey we walk impacts more than just ourselves; our attitudes, actions, and perceptions can touch everyone who sees a piece of themselves in our experiences. Our stories create ripples, connecting us across boundaries of fear, distance, and doubt.

This book is intended for those who feel unseen, misunderstood, or unsure of their next step. Navigating an unexpected diagnosis, wrestling with self-doubt, or searching for meaning after a major life change can feel overwhelming, and the challenges may seem insurmountable. The darkness can creep into every corner of our lives and suffocate us, leaving the path ahead in shadows and unclear.

I've been there.

Through my journey with the loss of a loved one, vision loss, chronic illness, and the challenges of finding my place in the world, I've learned that even in the darkest moments, light is always within reach. That light might not look like what you expected—it might flicker as a kind word is spoken, shimmer as you take a small step forward, or glow with the resilience you never realized you had. This book is here to remind you of that light, to help you uncover it, and to guide you as you find your way out of the darkness.

What You'll Learn

Through these pages, I'll share the lessons I've learned about navigating adversity, finding strength in community, and turning pain into purpose.

Together, we'll explore:

- **Self-advocacy:** How to advocate for your needs, trust your voice, and reclaim your power in a world that doesn't always listen.

- **Resilience through connection:** How to build a community that uplifts you and reminds you that you're not alone.

- **Purpose in adversity:** How to reframe life's challenges as opportunities to grow, inspire, and create meaningful change.

- **Breaking barriers:** How to challenge stereotypes, amplify underrepresented voices, and pave the way for others.

Why This Book Matters

I wasn't always comfortable sharing my story. When I was diagnosed with cone rod dystrophy, I felt like my world had shattered. After losing my vision and, later, living with debilitating chronic pain, I grieved for the life I thought I'd lost. But through the support of my community, the power of advocacy, and the strength I found within myself, I discovered that those cracks in my life weren't places of loss—they were openings where light could shine through.

This book is the culmination of those lessons, woven together through the stories and experiences that have shaped me. It's not a one-size-fits-all guide to overcoming adversity. Instead, it's an invitation to reflect, connect, and find your path forward.

Who This Book Is For

This book is for anyone who has felt lost, unseen, or uncertain. It's for those who are navigating the complexities of life with a disability, illness, or any unexpected challenge.

It's for people who want to build a more inclusive world and for those searching for hope in the face of hardship.

A Call to Action

Are you ready to uncover your light, embrace your journey, discover your strength, and take back your life? You already possess the power and the tools to make significant changes in your world. Let this book be your beacon. Let's take the first step together.

The Breaking Point

Struggle and Realizations

Finesse Literary Press Ltd.

1

Another Angel

Mini-Lesson: Loss teaches us about resilience and the unexpected strength within us.

The Day Everything Changed

IT WAS A COOL, crisp autumn day, bathed in sunlight—the kind of day that feels like a promise of something good. A Friday. Everything about it seemed perfect. I had a couple of precious hours to myself before picking up the kids from school. Treating myself, I brought home my favorite sushi, set it up at the living room coffee table, and turned on the TV. It was my moment of calm before the inevitable chaos of the afternoon.

Then, the knock came—loud and urgent, shattering the peace. At the door stood a police officer, his presence heavy with unspoken words. I watched his lips move, but it was as though the air had been sucked from the room, and I couldn't quite process what he was saying.

"Your mother has died," he said.

My heart dropped, and I struggled to comprehend his message.

He had no details, just a number for the coroner.

My mom had been away on a work trip. Questions swirled in my head, frantic and unrelenting. Had she been in an accident? She wasn't known for having a good sense of direction. Maybe she got lost? Was she ill? My mind clung to possibilities as I tried to grasp the impossible.

My mother is dead.

That day had started like any other, ordinary in its predictability. Yet by nightfall, my world was irrevocably changed.

The Weight of Absence

Loss, I've come to learn, is more than mere absence. It's the way that absence reverberates in the spaces where someone once was. It's the sound of laughter you no longer hear, the disrupted routines, and the void that lingers in the simplest moments. Losing my mom was the deepest pain I had ever known. It felt as though a piece of me had been torn away.

My relationship with my mom had gone through phases, but we had grown close in recent years. She adored my kids, showering them with the magnetic energy and laughter that defined her. She was blessed with a boundless ability to give and could light up a room simply by being in it. When she passed, the vibrant colors of my world faded into a grayscale haze of disbelief and heartache.

I struggled to comprehend how a vibrant fifty-eight-year-old woman could pass away alone in a hotel room. The coroner revealed that she'd gone to the hospital the day before, complaining of chest pain. They had found pneumonia in her lower left lung, ran some tests, and discharged her. She returned to her hotel room, fell asleep, and never woke up. My heart shattered as I flew to the hospital to see her lifeless body. Grief consumed me, leaving me lost in a fog of sorrow and unanswered questions.

The Shift Toward Resilience

In the days that followed, I wrestled with immense sadness and searched desperately for understanding. I questioned everything—life, purpose, and the path forward. *How do you move forward when someone who shaped your world is gone?* I didn't have an answer. All I could do was take one step at a time, even when each step felt impossibly heavy.

Grief forces us to look within ourselves and carve out a deeper understanding of our lives. In the quiet moments of reflection, I realized my mom had left me a gift—the courage to face the unknown. She had always been my anchor, and even in her absence, she taught me that resilience is about allowing ourselves to feel our pain rather than avoiding it, learning from it, and carrying its lessons forward.

I wrote her a letter, pouring out everything I wished I'd said. I read it aloud at her funeral, my voice trembling with pain but filled with raw honesty. It was the first time I had shared something so deeply personal in front of an audience. In those moments, my vulnerability became a source of strength, and I would carry that strength into the next chapter of my life.

Even now, over twenty years later, the pain can still feel unbearable. Yet, I keep moving forward, keeping her memory alive. Her life and her love have become my source of strength, reminding me that even in the face of immense hardship, there is light. It's not about erasing the pain but learning to coexist with it while seeking out moments of joy and purpose.

Finding Meaning in Loss

My mom's passing ignited a spark within me—a desire to live a life that honored her legacy of kindness and authenticity. Over time, I began to see how loss could be a teacher, showing me the value of connection and the importance of cherishing the moments we often take for granted.

One day, as I sifted through old photos of my mom and me, I thought about legacy. *What would it mean to live a life with purpose?* I didn't have the answers at the time. Beyond being a wife and mother, I had no idea what my purpose was. *What did I want to be remembered for?* It would be years before those answers were revealed, but even then, I knew it would mean stepping outside my comfort zone, embracing vulnerability, and turning my pain into purpose.

Grief isn't something to fix; it's something to carry. You can't just magically move on. Your parents may have modeled that stoic behavior or attitude toward loss, but avoiding our feelings can prolong the grieving process and lead to unhealthy behaviors. Ignoring how you feel or stuffing it away only weighs you down, leaving little space for truly living and moving forward.

I've come to realize that grief is not a weakness. It's love's natural response to loss. It comes in waves—sometimes sadness, sometimes anger, numbness, or longing—and there is no timeline for it. I've learned to give myself the space to feel and to sit with the grief rather than avoiding it. Grief is exhausting, and rest is part of the process.

Rediscovering life also takes time. We often need to reevaluate who we are in the wake of loss. We must find what brings us comfort or joy and allow ourselves to feel connected to others. To grieve is to honor the love you shared. To heal is to honor yourself. There's no rush. Be gentle as you take one step at a time.

***

Action Steps:

1. **Reflect on a Personal Loss**
   Take a moment to think about someone you've lost who profoundly impacted your life. What lessons or values did they leave behind? Write down a memory or story that captures their essence and how it continues to influence you.

2. **Identify a Way to Honor Their Memory**
   Choose one small action you can take to honor their legacy. This could be engaging in an act of kindness, pursuing a passion they encouraged, sharing their story, or simply taking a moment to reflect on their influence in your life.

3. **Embrace Vulnerability**
   Write a letter to your loved one expressing what you wish you could tell them now. If you feel ready, share it with someone close to you or keep it as a personal reflection of your journey through grief.

4. **Allow Space for Grief and Growth**

Acknowledge that grief is a process, not a destination. Give yourself permission to feel and process emotions without judgment. Identify one small step you can take this week to care for yourself as you navigate your journey.

By reflecting on loss, honoring the memory of your loved one, and embracing the lessons they taught, you can find strength in their legacy and continue to move forward with intention and resilience.

***

Closing Reflection

Loss has a way of breaking us open, but in those cracks, light can filter through. My mom's untimely passing was a defining moment for me, shaping how I approached the world and my role within it. Her legacy lives on in every bold step I take, every time I choose to see the good, and every time I extend compassion to someone who needs it. Her story didn't end with her passing; it continues to be written through the lives she touched—including mine.

In the years since my mom's passing, I've often drawn on the lessons grief taught me. I didn't know it then, but those lessons were preparing me for another trial—one that would challenge my strength and my roles as a caregiver and partner.

2

The Night That Redefined Us

Mini-Lesson: Resilience is not a solo act; it's a shared journey.

A Midnight Warning

Life has a way of lulling us into a sense of stability before everything changes. In the middle of the night on January 17, 2009, my husband's voice, low but laced with panic, pierced the quiet.

"I can't feel my hand," Tony said.

My heart pounded as I turned to him. Something wasn't right. I knew deep down what was happening, but my mind refused to accept it. His family had a history of strokes, and now, at just forty years old, it was happening to him.

The world around me slowed. I told myself I had to act. There wasn't time for fear.

"I'll drive you to the hospital," I said, trying to keep my voice steady.

"No," Tony slurred, his words barely intelligible. "I think I'm having a stroke. Call an ambulance."

The minutes that followed were a blur of frantic action—waking our daughter to watch for the paramedics, giving him aspirin in what I thought was an act of help but would later learn was a dangerous mistake for a hemorrhagic stroke.

When the paramedics arrived, their urgency confirmed my worst fear. Tony's blood pressure was dangerously high. They loaded him onto the stretcher, and I followed, climbing into the front seat of the ambulance. As we sped toward the hospital, the sirens reverberated through my chest. I sat frozen in silence, staring into the thick, cold fog of that January night, praying this wasn't the beginning of the end.

The First Long Night

The fluorescent lights of the ER cast an eerie glow as the ambulance pulled into Vancouver General Hospital. The paramedics wheeled Tony inside, and I followed close behind, rubbing my wedding band as if it were an anchor tethering me to reality.

In the neuro ICU, I stayed by his side, watching the machines beep and flash, their rhythm echoing the panic in my chest. The doctors worked to keep his blood pressure below 160, the level at which the blood vessel in his brain had burst. I clung to every word they said, trying to translate the medical jargon into something I could hold onto.

Tony drifted in and out of consciousness, mumbling occasionally. His frustration was palpable whenever the pulse oximeter taped to his finger slipped off. Every time it did, the incessant beeping filled the room, testing our patience.

I didn't sleep that night.

At 6:00 a.m., I called his boss. "Tony won't be coming into work today," I said, my voice cracking.

The truth was, I didn't know when—or if—he'd ever go back.

The Aftermath: Survival and Uncertainty

When the doctors confirmed that Tony had suffered a hemorrhagic stroke caused by hypertension, the air rushed from my lungs. *How could this happen?* He was young and healthy.

Tony spent seven days in the hospital. I was there for every moment, every test, and every uncertainty. But when he was discharged, the real journey began.

Just as I had found the strength to navigate life after my mother's death, I would now have to find a new reservoir of courage—this time as a caregiver to the man I loved.

Navigating a New Reality

At home, the adjustments were overwhelming, and exhaustion was relentless. Tony was determined to recover, to jog around the neighborhood, and get back to work. But the reality was far more complicated.

The strain of his recovery crept into every corner of our lives. I was a stay-at-home mom, raising three kids, and now I was also Tony's caregiver, driving back and forth to appointments, worrying over his comfort, and managing our home alone. At night, I lay awake, consumed by fear of what the future might hold.

Tony struggled, too. The fast-paced environment of his old job overwhelmed him. Tasks that once came naturally now felt impossible. Each failed attempt to return to normalcy brought frustration, self-doubt, and despair.

And yet, amidst the chaos, we began to redefine our roles. I became Tony's advocate, filling in the gaps when he couldn't find the words or didn't recognize the changes in himself. I was there for him and our children almost constantly, but in doing so, I lost sight of my own needs.

The Turning Point: Advocating for Ourselves

It took time—years, even—but we learned that resilience doesn't mean going it alone. It means leaning on each other and finding strength in the support of a community.

For Tony, that community came through the Semiahmoo House Society and the BC Brain Injury Association.

These groups gave him purpose, a sense of belonging, and the tools to rebuild his life in meaningful ways.

I returned to work, sometimes holding two to three jobs as I carried the weight of our family on my shoulders. It would take time—and another crisis—before I found my support system and a community to bolster me, but I came to realize that I was never truly alone.

Moments of Darkness: When It Felt Like Too Much

There were times when the cracks in our marriage felt like they might break us. Tony's explosive outbursts, my exhaustion, the kids' confusion all compounded into a heavy fog of despair.

We learned to seek outside help from therapists, family, and friends. Through therapy, family conferences, and countless difficult conversations, we began to rebuild— as individuals and as a team.

Becoming Each Other's Caregivers

Years later, when I faced my own health battles, Tony became my anchor. We discovered that caregiving is not a one-way street but a partnership.

***

Action Steps:

1. **Reflect on a time when life threw an unexpected challenge your way.**

   What changed in your life as a result?

   How did you adapt, and what strengths did you discover within yourself?

   Who or what helped you navigate that challenge?

2. **Now, consider one way you can offer similar support to someone in your life who may be**

facing their own storm.
Whether through a kind word, lending a hand, or simply being present, small acts of compassion can make a profound difference.

***

Closing Reflection

Adversity has a way of revealing what truly matters. It strips away the distractions and forces us to confront the core of who we are—as individuals, as partners, and as a family.

In the darkest moments, we found light. It wasn't easy, and it wasn't immediate, but it was there. That light became our guide, leading us forward, one step at a time.

As Tony and I navigated the uncharted waters of stroke recovery, caregiving, and redefining our relationship, we learned that resilience is not built in isolation. It is nurtured in the spaces where vulnerability is met with compassion and hardships are shared rather than shouldered alone. The stroke reshaped Tony's life and the fabric of our family, our roles, and the way we loved and supported each other. It taught us that survival requires adaptability, connection, and an unyielding belief in the power of love to heal. We would need these lessons for the next chapter in our lives—a journey that would challenge my strength in ways I never anticipated.

3

Blind Sighted: Seeing Beyond The Darkness

Mini-Lesson: True vision comes from understanding how to adapt and thrive.

AS CAREGIVERS, WE OFTEN focus so intensely on the needs of others that we forget to check in with ourselves. After Tony's stroke, I poured everything I had into supporting him, our children, and keeping our family afloat. But in the quiet moments, when the chaos subsided, I began noticing subtle signs of trouble in myself—signs I didn't yet understand. I could see, but I couldn't see. What started as a faint unease eventually grew into something I could no longer ignore. My vision was slipping away, and with it, my sense of who I was and how I would navigate the world.

The Diagnosis That Changed Everything

June 2015. The sun outside painted the day with warmth and light, but the office I sat in was dim and heavy with uncertainty.

"Cone rod dystrophy," the retinal specialist said. Three words that would alter the way I saw the world—and how the world would see me.

My mind felt numb, grasping for a way to come to terms with the implications of those three words, but failing. I asked her to write them down so I could make sense of them later.

Cone rod dystrophy is a rare, inherited retinal disease that slowly erases the retina's light-sensing cells. First, the cones, responsible for color and sharp central vision. Then, the rods, which govern peripheral vision and night sight.

There was no cure.

The diagnosis didn't feel real until I researched it on my phone while sitting on the bus. As the search results loaded, the truth began to unfold: my vision was slipping away, and there was nothing I could do to stop it.

The Long Road to Answers

Looking back, the signs had been there all along, buried in years of unexplained struggles.

As a child, I struggled to see the clock on the far wall of the classroom or read numbers on the overhead projector, even with thick glasses perched on my nose. My siblings also wore glasses, but no one questioned why I couldn't see as well as them.

In 2003, laser eye surgery offered me a temporary glimpse of a sharper, brighter world. For the first time, I could see clearly without glasses. I thought I had left my vision problems behind.

But within a few short years, things began to change. Night driving became terrifying. I couldn't see the lane lines, street signs, or license plates. Anxiety gripped me as I clung to the steering wheel, straining to see, and with my heart pounding.

I began to have difficulties, even in the daytime. I couldn't make out street signs until they were too close to be useful. License plates were just smudges in my vision.

Pedestrians appeared out of nowhere at crosswalks. My eyes struggled to adjust to changes in light, and I began to dread the dimming hours of dusk.

I went to the optometrist repeatedly, voicing my concerns. "I'm not seeing what I know I should be seeing." They ran their tests, but the results showed nothing wrong. Year after year, I left with a small prescription and mounting frustration.

The Decision to Stop Driving

By 2013, I knew I could no longer drive. The decision was excruciating. Driving represented independence, freedom, and responsibility for my family. But I couldn't ignore the danger I posed to myself and others.

Being unable to drive placed an enormous strain on my husband, Tony, who was still recovering from his stroke. We depended on my ability to travel to work, get to appointments, and get our children places. The decision to relinquish my license meant making considerable adjustments to how we functioned—and how I saw myself. As the primary breadwinner, I had taken on two to three jobs to keep us afloat. I was now navigating a world I could barely see, and it was terrifying.

Validation at Last

During a routine optometrist appointment in 2013, I impulsively decided to try contact lenses. My reasoning was simple: if I put the lenses directly on my eyes, maybe I'd see better. But the opposite happened; with the lenses on, my vision grew even blurrier.

That was the turning point. My optometrist finally recognized that there was a bigger problem and referred me to a retinal specialist.

When I met the specialist, I poured out years of frustration, fear, and doubt. Tearfully, I admitted that I felt like it was all in my head.

Her response was life-changing: "I believe you."

It would take two more years and a battery of tests before I had the answer I had been searching for—and dreading.

In June 2015, the diagnosis arrived. The relief of finally being heard clashed with the heartbreak of knowing my fears were real.

I was slowly going blind.

Living a Double Life

At the time I was diagnosed, I had just accepted a new job as a nursing assistant in a fertility clinic. It was an incredible opportunity—better hours, a shorter commute, and the financial stability my family desperately needed.

My family knew about my vision loss, but at work, I kept it a secret. I adapted through sheer determination. I memorized the layout of the procedure room, the placement of every tool, and the movements of my colleagues. Routine and muscle memory became my lifelines.

To my coworkers, I was meticulous and reliable, often praised for my attention to detail. No one suspected the anxiety that gnawed at me daily—the fear that someone would discover my secret.

Blindness, I learned, isn't always a visible and obvious disability. It exists on a spectrum, and I was navigating the liminal space between sighted and blind.

The First Steps Toward Acceptance

I struggled to cope for four years after my diagnosis before I finally reached out to CNIB (Canadian National Institute for the Blind) for help. Their support was a lifeline.

I began Orientation and Mobility training to learn how to use a white cane, particularly on public transit. But the stigma was heavy. I carried the cane but rarely used it, afraid of what people might think.

It took time, but I slowly understood that blindness wasn't the end of my story but the beginning of a new chapter. Slowly, I began to find my voice and advocate for myself. I disclosed my condition to HR and the doctors at work, terrified of their reactions. Instead, I was met with support and surprise. "You're the best we've ever had," they said.

Lessons in Vision

Living with vision loss has taught me that blindness is less about what you can't see and more about how you choose to adapt. It has shown me the power of visibility and the strength in being vulnerable.

My white cane, once a symbol of fear, has become a badge of pride. It represents my journey, my resilience, and my ability to navigate a world designed for sighted people.

***

Action Steps:

1. **Reflect on a challenge you've faced that required adaptation and resilience.**

   What changed in your life because of this challenge?

   What fears or doubts did you experience?

   What steps did you take—or could you take—to adapt and move forward?

2. **Next, commit to one tangible action:**

   If you're navigating a current challenge, identify a resource, tool, or person that can help support you, like a community group or professional guidance.

   If someone in your life is facing a similar challenge, reach out to offer encouragement or assistance.

By acknowledging your journey and taking proactive steps, you empower yourself to see beyond the obstacle and embrace the possibilities ahead.

***

Closing Reflection

Vision loss has redefined the way I see the world. It is no longer in terms of what I've lost but in what I've gained. It has opened doors to empathy, community, and self-discovery.

As I reflect on this journey, I have come to understand that true vision comes not from our eyes but from our ability to see beyond obstacles and embrace the possibilities that lie ahead.

As I came to terms with my vision loss, I gained a fragile sense of stability—a delicate balance where I could navigate life despite its challenges. I had adjusted to my limitations and found ways to keep moving forward for the sake of my family and myself. Yet, life has a way of unraveling even the most carefully held threads. Just when I believed I was regaining control, another unexpected challenge emerged, testing both my physical strength and the depths of my emotional and mental resilience.

4

Unrelenting Pain

Mini-Lesson: When life forces you to pause, it's an opportunity to reimagine your path.

A Day That Changed Everything

It was a new year with the promise of fresh beginnings. The air was crisp, the world was celebrating fresh starts, and resolutions hung in the air like unspoken promises. But for me, January 1, 2019 became the start of an unforeseen battle. The day began with an unrelenting throb on the right side of my head—a migraine-like headache that was unlike anything I had ever experienced.

I brushed it off as dehydration or stress, convinced it would fade. But the next morning, the headache was still there. And the next. And the next. What began as a single headache quickly unraveled into a relentless condition that would alter the course of my life.

Days turned into weeks.

Weeks into months.

The pain remained, constant and consuming. Every beat of my heart seemed to amplify the throbbing in my skull. By the time I received a diagnosis, I was so engulfed in darkness and pain that the name barely registered. *New Daily Persistent Headache*—a rare, chronic condition with no clear cause, no predictable path, and no cure.

The World Shrinking

For eight excruciating months, I was bedridden. The vibrant life I had so painstakingly struggled to build dissolved around me, replaced by the four walls of my bedroom, which felt like they were closing in more with every passing day.

I couldn't be the mother my children needed. I couldn't help with homework, make meals, or simply be present for them. I wasn't the partner my husband needed, either. Tony, still recovering from his health battles, bore the weight of our family responsibilities as I lay immobilized.

I felt useless. Broken.

My cellphone became my only connection to the outside world, but even that lifeline was fragile. Tasks as simple as ordering shampoo online became frustrating ordeals. Websites weren't designed with accessibility in mind. Product descriptions didn't exist. Buttons had no labels. I came face-to-face with the limitations of my vision loss, and each failure reminded me of how powerless I had become.

The Depth of Despair

The pain wasn't just physical—it seeped into every corner of my being. Depression arrived like a storm cloud, settling over me and whispering cruel lies:

You're a burden. You're worthless. Your family would be better off without you.

And for a time, I believed them.

I found myself grappling with questions of identity, purpose, and survival. There were days when I stared at the ceiling, too numb to cry and too broken to hope. I wondered if my children would even remember me as anything other than the ghost of a mother who barely existed.

But in the midst of the darkness, there was a flicker—a faint spark that refused to be extinguished. This difficult chapter of my life would soon reveal lessons about endurance, reinvention, and the extraordinary power of the human spirit.

Facing the Darkness

Pain medications and sleep provided some escape from my agony, and TV and my phone provided distraction when my pounding head could manage them. But when the distractions and escapes were gone, all that remained was me. I was forced to confront questions I had long avoided:

Who am I now?

What is left of me?

The answers didn't come all at once. Like pieces of a shattered mirror, they arrived in tiny, fragile fragments. Slowly, I began piecing them together. I couldn't control the pain, but I realized that I could control how I responded to it.

I started small. Sitting up in bed. Walking to the kitchen. Taking a shower. Each step was an act of rebellion against the pain that sought to consume me.

A Spark of Realization

Although a source of frustration, my phone became a tool for survival. As I struggled with inaccessible websites, anger began to replace despair.

Why were these barriers acceptable? Why was the world so inhospitable to people like me?

That anger became a spark, and that spark ignited a purpose.

I immersed myself in the world of digital accessibility. I learned about alt text, captioning, and inclusive design and wondered why more websites didn't use these tools. Deeply frustrated by the limitations I faced, I determined to change that for the blind and visually impaired community. My pain was no longer mine alone—it was shared by millions of others.

Action Through Advocacy

I took that anger and turned it into action, and soon discovered the power of advocacy. I began speaking out about the barriers I faced and connecting with others who shared my struggles. I opened an Instagram account, @purposeinview (Mok, 2020), to ensure my voice was heard. That account, and the community I built through it, became my lifeline.

With each post, I pushed for change, creating content that was as accessible as it was inspiring. I found purpose in amplifying voices like mine and advocating for a world where no one is left behind.

Lessons Learned

Living with NDPH has been a relentless challenge, but it has also been a teacher. It taught me that strength doesn't mean being unbreakable; it means finding ways to rise, even when everything feels impossible.

It taught me to look for joy in the smallest moments, to seek connection during isolation, and to redefine what it means to live a meaningful life.

***

Action Steps:

1. **Reflect on a time in your life when adversity forced you to pause and reevaluate your path.**

2. **Identify a Lesson Learned:** Write down one key insight or lesson you gained from that experience. What did it teach you about yourself, your strengths, or your priorities?

3. **Find Your Spark:** Think about a small action you can take to transform that lesson into purpose. It could be reaching out to someone for help, sharing your story to inspire others, or finding a community that resonates with your experience.

4. **Commit to Resilience:** Write one sentence of affirmation or intention to remind yourself of your ability to rise, adapt, and move forward—even in the face of challenges.

By taking these steps, you honor your journey and empower yourself to find light, even in the darkest moments.

***

Closing Reflection

Pain strips us bare, leaving us vulnerable and exposed. But it's in those moments of vulnerability when we sometimes find clarity. My journey with NDPH taught me that even in the darkest times, there is a spark of light. It may be faint, but it is enough to guide us forward.

This chapter of my life was one of struggle but also one of transformation. NDPH once again changed how I saw myself and the world, forcing me to pause, reflect, and reimagine my path. And while the pain remains, so does the spark. Sometimes, that spark is all we need to light the way.

As the relentless pain of NDPH forced me to confront my vulnerabilities, it also sparked an unexpected transformation. The challenges I faced sharpened my awareness of the barriers around me and awakened a deep desire to dismantle them. My struggles reshaped my perspective, showing me how a flicker of purpose could light the way forward.

During this time of introspection, a question began to form—a small, persistent thought that refused to fade: *What if there was a way to make the world more inclusive?* That question, simple yet profound, became the foundation for a new chapter of exploration and growth. In the midst of pain and uncertainty, I realized that the spark of curiosity could be the key to igniting change.

This question would lead me on a journey that would begin with a hesitant step into the world of social media—a step that would open doors to connection, advocacy, and transformation—and soon evolve into something far more significant, bridging communities and redefining what was possible.

The Turning Point

Growth and Advocacy

Finesse Literary Press Ltd.

5

Curiosity Leads to Change

Mini-Lesson: Change starts with asking the right questions and daring to take action.

The Birth of a Question

It started with a question—small and seemingly insignificant, yet powerful in its simplicity: *What if I tried?*

I had spent months in a haze, grappling with the pain of NDPH, adjusting to life with vision loss, and mourning the life I once had. I felt invisible, disconnected, and deeply isolated. I found myself at a crossroads. The physical and emotional trials of living with NDPH had stripped me bare, leaving me to confront who I was and what I wanted my life to stand for. While the pain remained constant, a flicker of curiosity began to grow within me. *What if this pain could lead to something greater?*

I realized that survival alone wasn't enough; I needed to find purpose. My mind turned to the untapped potential of connection, of using my experiences to create change for myself and for others navigating their own storms. This curiosity became my anchor as I wandered into a space I had always avoided: *social media.*

The idea felt ridiculous at first. Instagram, with its perfectly curated feeds, pristine aesthetics, and reliance on visuals, seemed like the last place for someone like me. What could I, a blind woman grappling with chronic illness, possibly offer in a world obsessed with appearances?

But the question lingered, stubborn and persistent: *What if I tried? What if Instagram could be something more than just a platform for polished images? What if I could challenge its limitations?*

I didn't know where the idea would lead me, but for the first time in a long time, I felt that spark of curiosity become an ember that refused to be extinguished.

Taking the First Step

In November 2020, I hesitantly created my account, @purposeinview[1]. My first post was raw and imperfect, a small introduction in a space that felt overwhelmingly vast.

I didn't have a strategy, a polished brand, or a clear sense of direction. But I had a mission: to connect, educate, and create a space where beauty and accessibility could coexist.

The learning curve was steep. When my pain would allow it, I spent hours researching hashtags, understanding algorithms, and deciphering what made a post resonate. Each like, comment, or share felt like a small victory, a reminder that someone out there was listening.

But there were moments of doubt, too. The first time I used an image description, I worried no one would notice or care. I wondered if my efforts to make my content accessible were worth it. Then, messages came from visually impaired followers, thanking me for the descriptions, which reignited my resolve.

Curiosity Turns to Connection

RESILIENCE AND PURPOSE

As I grew more comfortable with the Instagram platform, I began to see its potential as a tool for expression and a bridge between communities.

I started crafting image descriptions, adding alt text, and experimenting with audio captions. These small, thoughtful touches became a way to include the blind and visually impaired community in a space that had traditionally excluded them.

The messages I received reflected the impact of my efforts.

"I've never felt so seen in this space before."

"Thank you for making this accessible—it means so much."

These comments weren't just affirmations; they were fuel. They reminded me that advocacy didn't always have to be loud or grand. Sometimes, it was in the quiet details and the small efforts to make someone feel included.

A Ripple Effect

The connections I made through @purposeinview opened doors I hadn't even known existed. I started collaborating with brands, appearing on podcasts, and even delivering a TEDx talk. With each opportunity, I felt my life returning and my purpose becoming more evident. It was a different life than before, but it was a testament to the power of curiosity and daring to take the first step.

The community that formed around my account meant the most to me. Sighted followers began to ask questions about accessibility, eager to learn how they could be allies. The visually impaired community shared their stories, creating a tapestry of shared experiences and understanding.

This space became more than just an Instagram account. It became a movement.

Lessons in Learning

Through trial and error, I discovered the importance of showing up authentically. My posts weren't perfect, but they were real. I shared the messy parts of my journey, the frustrations, the triumphs, and everything in between.

I learned that advocacy wasn't about having all the answers; it was about asking the right questions and inviting others to join the conversation. It was about curiosity, growth, and a willingness to learn along the way.

***

Action Steps:

1. **Think of an area in your life where you've hesitated to take action because of doubt or fear.**

   Reflect on these questions:
   What if you tried? What small step could you take toward exploring this possibility?

   Who could benefit? How might your action create a ripple effect for yourself or others?

2. **Identify a simple, tangible step you can take to move closer to your goal or curiosity.**
   What's one thing you can do today?

Write down your answers, then commit to taking that first step—whether it's reaching out to someone for guidance, starting a project, or simply researching your idea.

Remember, big changes often start with small acts of courage.

***

Closing Reflection

Starting @purposeinview began as an act of curiosity, but it was also an act of courage. Change doesn't come from having everything figured out. It begins with a question, a willingness to try, and a commitment to keep learning.

That small spark of curiosity grew into a flame that illuminated my path and also the paths of those who joined me. Together, we created something meaningful—a space where curiosity led to connection, and connection led to change.

The spark that ignited my journey with @purposeinview opened doors to connection, advocacy, and change. It transformed an uncertain experiment into a platform of purpose, challenging stereotypes and inviting others into a more inclusive vision of the world. But as the platform grew, so did my realization of a deeper responsibility: the power of representation. I began to see how visibility could reshape narratives about how the world perceives disabilities, including blindness and visual impairment. This realization led me toward my next mission—to break down barriers through storytelling, collaboration, and advocacy, proving that representation changes everything.

6

Shifting Perceptions of Blindness

Mini-Lesson: Representation matters because it changes how the world sees us—and how we see ourselves.

The Power of Being Seen

As my journey with @purposeinview unfolded, I realized that my voice carried weight—not only as a storyteller, but as a representative of a broader community. Growing up, I rarely saw people like me reflected in the world around me. Blindness, when acknowledged at all, was either cloaked in stereotypes of helplessness or glorified with miraculous overachievement, leaving little room for the realities in between. This absence of nuanced representation became my motivation. As I began to share my journey with vision loss, I realized that my own perceptions of blindness were also changing. I began to question how I saw myself and how I assumed others saw me.

Could I, a blind woman, step into spaces where I didn't traditionally belong? Could I break barriers, challenge stereotypes, and show others like me that they, too, could take up space in the world?

The answers came, not all at once but in a series of small, determined steps.

I knew that visibility was more than being seen; it was about showing others, especially those navigating similar paths, that they belonged. It was time to challenge misconceptions and reimagine what inclusion could truly look like.

Making Accessibility Visible

I started @purposeinview with the mission of creating a space that was accessible to everyone. Instagram, a platform so rooted in visual content, felt like an ironic choice for someone losing their vision. But that was precisely the point. I wanted to challenge its limitations and make it more inclusive.

I started by adding detailed image descriptions to each post, weaving words that would invite blind and visually impaired followers to experience the content in their unique way.

As I experimented with alt text, audio descriptions, and reel captioning, I realized how much thought and effort was required to make content accessible. It wasn't an afterthought; it was an art. And it was worth it.

Every time I received a message from someone who felt included for the first time, it reaffirmed my mission. I wasn't just making content accessible; I was making people feel seen.

Advocacy in Every Step Forward

An unforgettable moment in my journey came from a message I received from across the globe. A young girl shared the joy and value of seeing someone who looked like her confidently navigating life with a white cane.

Her words stopped me in my tracks.

It cut through the noise of everyday life and reminded me why this work mattered so deeply. She shared how my accessible Instagram images made her feel less alone and more empowered to embrace her identity.

This poignant connection ignited a determination within me to ensure that representation wasn't just an occasional breakthrough but a consistent, visible reality. It reaffirmed my belief that every photo, every piece of content, and every collaboration held the potential to break barriers, shift perceptions, and create meaningful change. Fashion became a vehicle for that advocacy—a way to challenge assumptions about blindness and redefine what inclusion looks like.

The message from the young girl reminded me that advocacy goes beyond visibility to connection and impact. As I continued to share my story, I realized that each post, image, and word could ripple outward, creating opportunities for representation and collaboration.

Breaking Barriers Through Collaboration

Collaboration became a cornerstone of my advocacy journey, opening doors to create meaningful change.

It began with Aille Design[1] (Aille Design, 2025), a brand that reimagines fashion through tactile Braille elements. After placing an order for one of their custom products, they featured my story on their Community Blog, where I shared the vision behind @purposeinview. That blog post became a catalyst, connecting me to brands and organizations eager to redefine inclusion. What began as a personal journey evolved into a collective effort to break barriers, one collaboration at a time.

It was through that blog post that Purdys Chocolatiers discovered me, leading to my involvement in their groundbreaking Braille Holiday Box[2] campaign. Designed in consultation with the blind and visually impaired community, the box was a first of its kind, featuring Braille orientation tabs, a Braille chocolate legend, and a QR code linking to a screen-reader-friendly version. It exemplified the possibilities of inclusive design.

Specsavers Canada[3] invited me to speak about eye health while showcasing their stylish frames, breaking the stereotype that blind people don't wear glasses or can't be fashionable. It was empowering to demonstrate how fashion and functionality can coexist and challenge misconceptions about blindness.

These partnerships in representation pushed boundaries. Some collaborations were effortless, with teams already invested in accessibility. Others required hard conversations, where I had to explain why accessibility wasn't a luxury but a necessity. These collaborations and partnerships became opportunities to educate and inspire their audience about the importance of accessibility.

Each alliance has been a step toward changing perceptions and showing that inclusion can be transformative. Together, we've broken barriers, proving that when advocacy and innovation intersect, the impact is limitless.

Lessons in Advocacy

These collaborations taught me that advocacy isn't always about grand gestures. Sometimes, it is in the small, everyday choices we make to include others. It is in the language we use, the stories we tell, and the spaces we create.

I was reminded again of the power of vulnerability. Sharing my story wasn't easy—it meant opening myself up to scrutiny, judgment, and misunderstanding. But it also created a space for connection. When I was honest about my struggles, it permitted others to be honest about theirs.

Advocacy, I realized, wasn't about being perfect. It was about showing up, speaking out, and being willing to learn.

Representation Changes Everything

As my platform grew, so did my understanding of the importance of representation. Being seen as a blind woman on stage, in fashion campaigns, or leading conversations about accessibility was more than a personal goal. It was about the countless people watching—people who needed to know that they, too, could belong in these spaces.

Representation sparks a ripple effect. When one person steps forward, it opens the door for countless others to follow, challenging entrenched perceptions and reshaping narratives.

***

Action Steps:

1. **Reflect on Representation in Your Life:** Consider an area in your life—whether at work, at school, or within your community—where diverse representation is missing. Ask yourself:

   Who is not being seen or heard?

   What barriers might exist for them?

2. **Identify a Step Toward Inclusivity**: Choose one tangible action you can take to foster greater inclusivity in that space. Examples include:

   a. Advocating for accessible resources like captions, alt text, or Braille materials.

   b. Amplifying underrepresented voices by sharing their stories or ideas.

   c. Encouraging others to challenge stereotypes through education and conversation.

3. **Start a Ripple Effect:** Commit to one specific way you can spark change today. Whether it's having a discussion about accessibility, incorporating inclusive practices into your work, or creating a space for underrepresented voices, remember that even small actions can create ripples of change.

4. **Share Your Impact:** Document your efforts and share what you've learned with others. By doing so, you inspire others to take steps toward inclusivity.

Reminder: Advocacy and representation begin with one small, intentional act. By taking this step, you contribute to a more inclusive world where everyone feels seen, valued, and empowered to thrive.

***

Closing Reflection

Shifting perceptions of blindness started with a single question: *What if I tried?* That question led to a platform, a mission, and a movement. It taught me that representation isn't just about visibility—it's about possibility.

When we dare to step into the light, we shift how the world perceives us and how we perceive ourselves. That shift is the foundation of representation—and the first step toward building a more inclusive world.

Representation has shown me the power of visibility to challenge stereotypes and rewrite the narrative around blindness and disability. Through my collaborations and storytelling, I began to see that advocacy could create ripples far beyond individual impact. Each step forward and every connection made proved that when we break down barriers, we pave the way for others to follow. Yet, as I reflected on this journey, I realized that true inclusion required more than visibility. It demanded systemic change—especially in areas like education, technology, and employment, where accessibility is often an afterthought. The next step in my journey was about ensuring that everyone has the tools and opportunities to thrive.

7

Breaking Barriers: Accessibility as a Path to Empowerment

Mini-Lesson: Accessibility is more than inclusion; it's about unlocking potential.

The World Isn't Designed for Everyone

When I was first diagnosed with cone rod dystrophy, I didn't fully grasp what it would mean for my daily life.

While adjusting to vision loss, I learned that I would have to navigate a world that wasn't designed with me in mind. From educational tools to employment practices, accessibility was often an afterthought, if it was considered at all.

Accessibility is a moral imperative and a practical necessity. It is more than a tool for inclusion; it is the key to unlocking potential for individuals like me and entire communities and industries. Without it, doors remain closed, and talent goes untapped.

Barriers in Education and Employment: Attitudinal Barriers

The Invisible Weight of Stigma

One of the hardest things about losing my vision wasn't the physical adjustments—it was the psychological battle. I struggled with the loss of self-confidence, self-belief, and self-image that came with the idea of using a white cane. To me, the cane was the ultimate symbol of blindness and all the negative connotations I had about vision loss. In my mind, being blind meant being different. That difference felt like a glaring vulnerability I couldn't escape.

I live in Vancouver, a city celebrated for its diversity, and yet, in all my years here, I had never seen anyone like me—a blind Asian woman navigating the world with a white cane. Even though I was raised in a Westernized way, cultural influences lingered. In many Asian cultures, disability is often a quiet, hidden reality. It isn't openly discussed, and the silence around it can be isolating. Without visible representation, I felt like I was stepping into uncharted territory alone.

This lack of representation shaped how I saw myself. It amplified the stigma in my head, the fear of how the world would perceive me, and the doubt that I could belong in spaces I had once moved through with ease.

Representation and the Power of Empowering Interactions

Self-esteem and self-belief are built through experiences, interactions, and reflections of ourselves in the world. When those reflections are absent, it can feel like there's no place for you. That's why representation matters so profoundly—not just in media or campaigns but in everyday life.

Imagine if, while growing up, I had seen other blind Asian women confidently navigating life with a white cane. How would my perception be different if I had been introduced to stories of disability as part of the broader human experience instead of something to be pitied or hidden? Those empowering interactions could have shifted my understanding of myself and the world.

I kept coming back to this question: *How can I be that empowering experience for someone else?*

Shifting the Narrative

Accessibility isn't just about compliance or convenience; it's about creating a world where everyone can succeed. It's about creating spaces, both physical and digital, where everyone feels like they belong. Digital accessibility, in particular, is essential to equity and inclusion in the modern world.

Making content accessible is more than just a strategy for businesses to create stronger brand presence or improved customer experiences (though it undeniably does both). Above all, it's the right thing to do.

Technology can level the playing field in ways that were unimaginable a generation ago. As one of 1.2 million

Canadians living with vision loss, I've experienced firsthand how transformative accessible technology can be. Accessible tools, content, and opportunities aren't just convenient—they're a necessity.

Breaking Down Barriers

As I grew into my identity as a blind person, I realized that the stigma I had internalized was both a personal battle and a societal one. Attitudinal barriers aren't simply the assumptions others make about us; they're the stories we come to believe about ourselves.

It took time and courage, but I began to see my white cane differently. Instead of being a symbol of vulnerability, it was a symbol of strength, independence, and resilience. I wasn't hiding anymore. By stepping into the world as my authentic self, I challenged my own perceptions and the perceptions of everyone around me.

This realization fueled my advocacy. From the stigma surrounding disability to the barriers ingrained in systems, it became clear to me that change was both necessary and possible. Through creating accessible content on Instagram, speaking at events, and partnering with organizations, I was determined to help shift the narrative around blindness and disability.

***

Action Steps:

1. **Reflect on Barriers in Your Own Spaces**
   Identify one space in your life—in your workplace, school, or digital community—where accessibility or inclusion is lacking. Consider both physical and attitudinal barriers.

   Are there practices or norms that unintentionally exclude others?

   Are there voices or perspectives missing?

2. **Take One Action to Foster Accessibility**
   Choose a tangible step you can take to address these gaps.

   a. Advocate for changes in policy or design to

make the space more inclusive.

b. Amplify the voices of individuals who have been underrepresented or excluded.

c. Educate yourself and others about accessibility tools, like screen readers or alt text, and implement them in your sphere of influence.

3. **Challenge Stigma Through Awareness**
Reflect on any assumptions you might hold—about yourself or others—that reinforce barriers. Replace them with empowering actions, such as:

a. Sharing a personal story that highlights the importance of accessibility.

b. Supporting others in challenging stereotypes within your community.

4. **Empower the Next Generation**
Look for ways to become a role model or ally for those navigating similar barriers. Representation matters at every level, and your actions can create a ripple effect of inclusion and empowerment.

5. **Commit**

   Write down your action plan, including one step you will take this week to foster accessibility, and revisit it regularly to track progress. Change starts with a singlestep, and your commitment can inspire others to follow.

***

Closing Reflection

Attitudinal barriers are often invisible, but their impact can be profound. By challenging stereotypes and fostering representation, we can begin to break them down—for ourselves and for the generations that follow. When accessibility becomes a priority and inclusion is standard practice, we unlock the potential that lies within us all.

As my journey into advocacy deepened, I began to understand the profound connection between accessibility and representation. Accessibility ensures that we can participate; representation ensures that we belong. My work in education, technology, and employment illuminated how systemic barriers keep people with disabilities on the margins. But breaking those barriers was only part of the solution. To truly create change, we needed to shift how people saw disability—from a limitation to a rich, multidimensional experience.

This realization brought me to the heart of my next chapter: the power of being seen. Representation is about redefining narratives and creating space for others to see themselves reflected in places they've historically been excluded. Whether on a TEDx stage, in the pages of a book, or through a social media post, I discovered that sharing my story and representing my community had the power to challenge stereotypes, inspire inclusion, and ignite change.

The Empowered Point

Connection and Representation

Finesse Literary Press Ltd.

8

Representation

Mini-Lesson: To be seen is to be empowered. To represent others is to make change possible.

The Power of Being Seen

Representation is the bridge between being seen and being understood. As I embraced my identity as a blind content creator and advocate and began sharing my journey with vision loss, I realized representation is not just about breaking barriers for ourselves; it's about opening doors for others, changing perceptions, and building pathways for change. It is an act of empowerment. When we step into spaces where we've historically been excluded, we say to the world,

We belong here, too.

Standing on the TEDx Stage

I stood on the TEDx stage, prepared to do more than give a speech. I was there to shatter stereotypes, redefine perceptions, and inspire a new vision of what inclusion truly means. Titled *Blind Sighted*, my talk was a culmination of my journey: a blend of personal reflection, advocacy, and a call to action.

For several years, I had wrestled with the invisible barriers of disability—societal stigmas, internalized self-doubt, and a lack of representation. The absence of representation in my life whispered to me that my story didn't belong in the larger narrative. But on that stage, I decided to change that narrative, for myself and for countless others who feel unseen, unheard, and unrepresented.

Shattering the Glass

I opened with a memory—one that had profoundly shaped me. At three years old, sitting on the carpet of our family home, I heard the sound of glass shattering around me. Someone had thrown a rock through our window in a cruel act of exclusion and rejection of my family's Asian heritage. That moment was my first encounter with feeling different and the beginning of understanding that not everyone sees belonging as a universal right.

The metaphor of shattered glass carried through my talk, symbolizing both the breaking of old perceptions and the opportunity to reassemble those fragments into something new and meaningful.

A Lens of Accessibility

I invited the audience to join me in seeing the world through an accessible-first lens. I shared how, as a blind woman, tools like my smartphone become more than a means of connection but also allow for greater independence—a flashlight, a wallet, a GPS navigator, and a lifeline to the sighted world. I revealed how social media became a gateway for building community, amplifying voices, and breaking barriers.

Social media, a space historically dominated by visuals, was where I first dared to challenge convention. Through accessible content—alt text, image descriptions, and captions—I connected the sighted and visually impaired communities, fostering understanding and collaboration.

Representation Matters

The heart of my talk was a simple but profound message: representation changes everything. I wanted the audience to know that blindness is a spectrum—that blind individuals use cell phones, cook meals, put on makeup, and lead full lives. Stereotypes reduce us to one-dimensional characters, but representation expands those dimensions, creating space for complexity, diversity, and authenticity.

I spoke of the importance of social inclusion, quoting the United Nations Convention on the Rights of Persons with Disabilities: "Disability results from the interaction between persons with impairments and attitudinal and environmental barriers that hinder their full and effective participation in society."[1]

By addressing those barriers—both physical and attitudinal—we can build a world where no one feels excluded.

A Call to Action

As I concluded, I held up a metaphorical mirror, challenging the audience to see themselves in the story of inclusion. I asked them to reflect on their biases and their role in creating or dismantling barriers.

Bravely exposing my vulnerability, I shared how I learned to embrace my white cane, an outward symbol of blindness I once feared. Instead of seeing it as a mark of difference, I now view it as a bridge—an emblem of independence, resilience, and connection.

My final words were not just an ending but an invitation:

"When we look in the mirror and see a reflection of ourselves, let's shatter the glass to see beyond that reflection to the inclusive and diversely connected community we truly are. When we start to look at digital accessibility through an accessible-first lens, no one will be left out or left behind."

Becoming an Author: Echoes of Grace and Strength

When Sabine Kvenberg invited me to contribute to her anthology, *Become Empowered: Echoes of Grace and Strength*[2], I felt both honored and apprehensive. Writing my story opened a window to my vulnerabilities, fears, and triumphs. Through this writing process, I discovered the power of storytelling—a force capable of inspiring change, fostering connection, and challenging perceptions.

Writing My Truth

My chapter, *Blind Sighted,* starts with three words that changed my life forever: *cone rod dystrophy*. These words signaled the decline of my vision, but they also marked the beginning of a journey of transformation. As I wrote about that fateful day in June 2015, when my retinal specialist delivered the diagnosis, I found myself reliving every moment—the fear, the questions, and the heavy burden of uncertainty.

The act of writing allowed me to piece together the fragments of my story, showing how each challenge I faced shaped me into the person I am today. It was an opportunity to give voice to my experiences with vision loss, struggles with self-acceptance, and my determination to create a life filled with meaning and purpose.

Representation Through Words

I realized that sharing my story, while beneficial to me, was more about creating visibility for others in the blind and visually impaired community. In our society, narratives of disability are often limited to either extreme struggle or extraordinary triumph. I wanted my words to represent the nuanced, messy, and beautiful reality of living with vision loss.

For someone who grew up without seeing individuals like myself reflected in books, media, or society, contributing to *Become Empowered: Echoes of Grace and Strength* was a profound moment of representation. My story became a mirror for those who, like me, felt unseen. Blindness is a spectrum that comes with challenges and victories, and it is just one part of a whole and vibrant identity.

Breaking Stereotypes and Barriers

Writing also gave me the chance to address common misconceptions about blindness. In my chapter in Kvenberg's book (Kvenberg, 2024), I emphasized that blindness doesn't always look the way people expect. Many blind individuals, like myself, capably navigate the world with the help of tools like white canes, assistive technology, or guide dogs. Yet, we often face attitudinal barriers—assumptions that we are incapable, dependent, or unworthy of opportunities.

I sought to break down those barriers through sharing my personal and professional journey. From working as a nursing assistant to becoming an advocate, a blind content creator, a TEDx speaker, and now an author, I aimed to show the richness and possibility of life beyond sight.

The Ripple Effect of Storytelling

One of the most rewarding aspects of becoming an author has been hearing from readers who found pieces of themselves in my words. Some were parents seeking hope after their child was newly diagnosed with vision loss. Others were individuals with disabilities who felt empowered to share their stories.

Storytelling has a ripple effect. By sharing my truth, I honored my journey and opened a door for others to step through and claim their narratives. *Become Empowered: Echoes of Grace and Strength* is a tapestry of voices, with each thread contributing to a larger story of resilience, growth, and empowerment.

Each time I've shared my story, I've seen the ripple effect of representation. It's in the messages from people who feel less alone. It's in the conversations that spark new perspectives. And it's in the growing awareness that inclusion isn't optional—it's essential.

A Call to Action

Writing reinforced my belief that representation matters. When we share our stories, we create pathways for others to follow. To anyone considering whether their voice deserves to be heard, I say this: Your story has the power to inspire, connect, and create change.

Through writing, I found a greater purpose—to ensure that no one feels alone in their struggles and that everyone knows they have the strength to overcome. Together, our stories can reshape how the world sees disability and, most importantly, how we see ourselves.

Breaking Stereotypes and Barriers

Through TEDx, *Become Empowered: Echoes of Grace and Strength*, and my advocacy work, I've learned that representation is about showing up authentically. It's about dismantling stereotypes and breaking down barriers, one story at a time.

I've often been told that I don't "look blind." It's a comment steeped in misconception, and it speaks to the narrow lens through which society views disability. Every time I step into a space—whether on stage, in a book, or through my social media platforms—I'm showing that blindness exists on a spectrum and isn't the same for everyone.

Representation challenges the assumptions people have about disabilities. It expands the narrative and creates space for the diverse experiences of people with disabilities. It's not just about being visible; it's about being part of the change that makes visibility possible for others.

***

Action Steps:

1. **Reflect on Representation in Your Life**
   Think back to a time when you felt truly seen or represented—whether in your community, workplace, or through a story that resonated with you.

How did it make you feel?

What impact did it have on your confidence, sense of belonging, or ability to take action?

2. **Identify Opportunities for Representation**
Look for areas in your life or work where representation is missing or voices are underrepresented.

Is there a story or perspective that needs to be shared?

Are there individuals who could benefit from a platform or moment of visibility?

3. **Take a Tangible Step Toward Empowerment**
Commit to one action that fosters representation in your sphere of influence.

   a. Share your own story or amplify the voices of others through conversations, social media, or public forums.

   b. Advocate for inclusive practices in your community or workplace, such as celebrating diverse narratives or creating mentorship opportunities.

c. Design resources, campaigns, or initiatives that reflect and include a broad spectrum of experiences.

4. **Foster Inclusive Representation**
Work to break down stereotypes by showcasing authenticity and diversity in the spaces you inhabit. Challenge narrow narratives and make room for complexity and nuance in how people are represented.

5. **Commit to Ongoing Advocacy**
Representation is not a one-time effort—it's a continual process of creating space for others to be seen and heard. Write down one goal you can work toward in the coming months to make representation a consistent priority in your advocacy, work, or community engagement.

By reflecting on your own experiences and taking actionable steps, you can create moments of empowerment that ripple outward, fostering a more inclusive and understanding world.

***

Closing Reflection

Representation is more than being visible—it's about creating connections, challenging assumptions, and opening doors. When we dare to be seen, we make it possible for others to do the same. Together, we can redefine what inclusion looks like and build a world where everyone feels empowered to take up space regardless of ability.

Seeing ourselves reflected in the world is both a personal victory and a collective step toward creating a more inclusive society. Representation transforms barriers into bridges, permitting others to imagine their place in spaces where they've historically been excluded. It's a powerful ripple effect that begins with a single voice but resonates far beyond.

As I reflect on my journey of representation, I am naturally led to a deeper exploration of milestones that once felt unattainable. From standing on stages to collaborating with inspiring communities, each achievement has shown me that the seemingly impossible can become reality with courage, connection, and belief in our potential. The next step is to reflect on how these goals, once out of reach, became catalysts for transformation and symbols of what is possible when we dare to dream.

9

I Can Achieve That

Mini-Lesson: Goals that once seemed impossible can become reality with the right mindset and support.

THERE'S A DISTINCT MOMENT when a dream shifts from something intangible—hovering just out of reach—to a milestone firmly within your grasp. It doesn't happen all at once. For me, it was a series of steps, each fueled by equal parts vulnerability, determination, and the support of those who believed in me when I struggled to believe in myself. At the heart of every achievement was a tiny light—the unwavering belief that I was capable of more, even when doubt whispered otherwise.

As I look back on my journey, I see a trail of milestones—some small, others monumental—that mark my growth. From the first shaky steps of public speaking to representing global brands, I've learned that each achievement is more than an endpoint; it's a foundation for the next possibility. These moments have taught me that the impossible isn't a fixed barrier; it's an invitation to explore what could be with the right mindset and a willingness to try.

Overcoming Self-Doubt

Self-doubt is a powerful force that often took up residence in my mind. *Could I, a woman navigating vision loss, stand on a stage, mentor others, or represent a global brand?* These questions loomed large, but I realized the answers would only come if I dared to try.

One of the first challenges I faced was public speaking. It was a personal hurdle that felt like an act of rebellion against every fear I'd carried about being seen and heard. Standing before an audience for the first time, I shared my story with trembling hands and a quivering voice, but the reaction from the crowd was one of warmth and connection. They didn't just see my vision loss—they saw me.

That moment was transformative, showing me that my voice had power and my story could inspire.

Becoming a Bold Blind Beauty Ambassador

Joining the *Bold Blind Beauty*[1] community marked another pivotal step in my journey. When I was first diagnosed with cone rod dystrophy, I turned to the internet in search of stories—narratives of people living and thriving with vision loss. I discovered *Bold Blind Beauty* and began reading about women and men who were navigating life with vision loss while breaking barriers. Their stories inspired me deeply and gave me hope at a time when I felt lost.

Years later, as I established myself on social media, I experienced a full-circle moment: I became an ambassador for *Bold Blind Beauty*. Being part of this community of strong, resilient people felt like coming home. Like me, they were breaking barriers and challenging stereotypes. Representing *Bold Blind Beauty* was a wonderful opportunity for advocacy, redefining beauty standards, and showing that blindness is not a limitation but a rich and meaningful facet of diversity.

As an ambassador, I had the opportunity to share my experiences and insights with an audience eager to learn about accessibility, representation, and inclusion. Each conversation reinforced a powerful truth: my lived experiences were valuable—and even more, they were essential. Together, we amplified the message that beauty and strength come in many forms and that inclusivity enriches everyone.

Mentorship with Jillian Harris

From the moment I enrolled in Jillian Harris' *The Jilly Academy*[2], I knew it would be a transformational journey. Jillian Harris, a celebrated designer and entrepreneur, embodies creativity, compassion, and connection—qualities I deeply admire and aspire to incorporate into my own work and community.

The Jilly Academy, a three-course business masterclass designed for entrepreneurs, influencers, and marketers, offered far more than lessons in branding and storytelling. It provided me with tools to amplify my voice while staying rooted in authenticity. Through the courses, I learned to lean into my truth, share my unique perspective unapologetically, and recognize my lived experiences as a source of strength. Jillian's insights became a rallying call to embrace my identity and purpose with conviction.

Becoming a member of *The Jilly Academy* alumni was one of the most enriching aspects of joining this vibrant community. The connections I made offered invaluable support, camaraderie, and shared learning. At the first anniversary of *The Jilly Academy*, I entered and won a speaking contest. The prize included funding for my business as well as a one-on-one session with Jillian, where we focused on using my voice as a public speaker. This session was an incredibly affirming experience. Jillian believed in my vision and encouraged me to dream even bigger.

Another standout experience was being featured on Jillian's blog, *A Candid Conversation with Alumni Member Anne on Finding Purpose in Entrepreneurship*[3]. In the feature, I reflected on my mission to make beauty and connection accessible to everyone, regardless of ability. Jillian's team shared my story with her vast audience, shining a light on my work with @purposeinview and the values I strive to represent.

Being part of *The Jilly Academy* equipped me with skills to navigate business and social media, but more importantly, it illuminated how I could create impact and leave a legacy. It inspired me to focus on the soul of my work—connecting deeply with my audience while staying true to my vision and values.

Jillian often says, "Connect, communicate, and then create." These words have become a guiding principle in my life. I've learned that success isn't just about achievements; it's about the relationships we build and the ripples of change we inspire.

Now, as I stand on stages, form meaningful partnerships, and pursue dreams I once thought unattainable, I carry the lessons Jillian instilled: dream boldly, lead with kindness, and never underestimate the power of your own story.

Celebrating Milestones

Each of these experiences marked a milestone in my journey—moments where I could look back and say, "I achieved that." More than just accomplishments, they were affirmations of my growth, my resilience, and the support system that carried me through.

Each achievement was a step toward a larger vision: to create a world where everyone feels seen, valued, and empowered to chase their dreams.

A New Perspective on Possibility

As I reflect on these milestones, I'm reminded that impossible goals become attainable when approached with the right mindset and support. Surrounding myself with mentors, allies, and a community that believes in my potential has been transformative.

The power to achieve is not reserved for the extraordinary—it's something we all possess, waiting to be unlocked by courage, curiosity, and connection. The barriers you face today don't have to define your tomorrow. Embrace those moments of transformation and the lessons they bring so you, too, can look back and say, "I achieved that."

***

Action Steps:

1. **Reflect on Moments of Representation**
   Think about a time when you felt seen or represented in your life.

How did it impact your confidence, sense of belonging, or ability to take action?

What emotions did it evoke, and how did it shape your perspective?

2. **Identify Gaps in Representation**
Consider the spaces where representation is still missing or where diverse voices are underrepresented in your life, workplace, or community. Are there stories that need to be shared or perspectives that need amplification?

Who in your sphere of influence could benefit from visibility or support?

3. **Take Intentional Action**
Commit to one concrete action that fosters representation:

   a. Share your personal story or amplify someone else's story through social media, conversations, or public platforms.

   b. Advocate for representation in media, workplace practices, or community initiatives.

c. Collaborate on projects that celebrate diversity and inclusivity.

4. **Challenge Stereotypes and Foster Belonging**
Work to dismantle narrow narratives about marginalized communities:

a. Educate yourself on the lived experiences of others.

b. Create opportunities for authentic and diverse voices to take center stage.

c. Be an ally who actively supports inclusion and representation.

5. **Commit to Ongoing Advocacy**
Representation is not a one-time event; it requires consistent effort. Write down a goal to sustain your commitment to fostering inclusion, whether through mentorship, advocacy, or storytelling. Revisit and refine this goal as you continue your journey.

By taking these steps, you can create a ripple effect that empowers others to feel seen, valued, and understood. Together, we can create a world where representation isn't the exception but the norm.

***

Closing Reflection

Every milestone begins with a single step. With the right mindset, the willingness to try, and the support of a community that believes in you, there's no limit to what you can achieve.

Reflecting on the milestones I've achieved, I realize that none of them happened in isolation. Behind every breakthrough moment was a foundation built on love, resilience, and the strength of the relationships that have supported me. My journey has been as much about finding my own voice as it has been about leaning on those who have walked beside me. At the heart of this support is Tony, my husband and partner through life's most challenging seasons. Our story is one of caregiving and overcoming adversity, and especially about the evolution of a partnership that has weathered storms and emerged stronger. Before I could stand on stages or build a platform, I first had to learn what it means to truly be seen, supported, and loved. This is the story of how we became each other's caregivers and what it taught us about resilience, connection, and the depths of love.

10

Becoming Each Other's Caregivers

Mini-Lesson: Love and partnership mean holding space for each other's growth, even in adversity.

RELATIONSHIPS ARE OFTEN PAINTED as fairy tales, but the reality of love—true, enduring love—is far more complicated. The deeper and more personal narrative is in the shared struggles, unspoken sacrifices, triumphs, and moments of mutual support. My relationship with my husband, Tony, has been defined by this kind of love. As our lives evolved, so did our roles within it. Love is not static; it adapts, bends, and grows with life's challenges. For Tony and me, those challenges taught us what it truly means to care for one another—in action and in spirit.

When we first met, we were partners in the simplest sense—sharing the joys and challenges of life side by side. But life has a way of testing relationships, throwing unexpected storms into calm waters. For us, the first storm came in 2009, when Tony suffered a stroke.

Learning to Care

In an instant, our roles shifted. Tony, my strong, dependable partner, became a survivor. And I, unprepared but determined, became his caregiver. The weeks and months that followed were a blur of doctor's appointments, rehabilitation sessions, and sleepless nights, grieving the life we had lost and figuring out a new normal. I had to learn how to advocate for him in medical settings, manage our household, and hold our family together.

It was one of the hardest periods of our lives. At times, I questioned whether we would make it as a couple and as a family. The stroke brought changes to Tony's personality, leaving me wondering if I was talking to the man I married or "stroke Tony." Yet, despite these challenges, I saw his resilence as he worked tirelessly to regain his independence. He pushed through physical and emotional barriers with determination, inspiring me every step of the way.

But caregiving is not without its toll. There were moments when the weight of responsibility felt unbearable. I would cry into my pillow at night, feeling both helpless and guilty for my exhaustion. Yet, even in my lowest moments, our children reminded me why we were fighting so hard—for each other and for them.

The Roles Reverse

A decade later, life tested us again. My vision loss from cone rod dystrophy progressed after my 2015 diagnosis. Then, in 2019, I was diagnosed with NDPH, a chronic headache condition that left me bedridden for months. Suddenly, Tony was thrust into the role of caregiver, navigating unfamiliar waters as he supported me through pain and depression.

Watching him step into this role with grace and compassion was humbling and heartbreaking. He managed everything—our home, our family—all while continuing to cope with the lingering effects of his stroke. I knew it wasn't easy for him. Just as I had once felt the weight of caregiving, he now carried that same burden.

Holding Space for Growth

These challenging seasons taught us that caregiving isn't as much about doing as it is about *being*. It's about holding space for each other's pain without trying to fix it and offering support without diminishing autonomy. It's about listening, even when there are no words to make things better.

We also learned the importance of self-care. As much as we wanted to give everything to each other, we realized we couldn't pour from an empty cup. Tony found solace in gardening and working at a golf course, while I found moments of peace through storytelling and connecting with my online community. These small acts of self-care became vital in sustaining our strength for one another.

Resilience Through Love

If there's one thing our journey has taught us, it's that love is resilient. It bends but doesn't break, adapts but doesn't falter. It's not about who gives and who receives but about the mutual understanding that we're in this together.

Our relationship has evolved through caregiving. We've seen each other at our most vulnerable, and these moments of raw honesty have strengthened our bond. We've learned to celebrate small victories—a good day, a shared laugh, a quiet moment of peace—because those are the threads that weave a life worth living.

As Tony and I navigated the uncharted waters of caregiving, we learned profound lessons about trust, resilience, and advocacy. Supporting each other through life's most challenging moments required us to speak up—for each other and sometimes for ourselves. These experiences illuminated a simple yet powerful truth: advocacy is an act of love for others and ourselves.

Lessons in Partnership

Caregiving taught us that partnership is not about perfection; it's about showing up, day after day, even when it's hard. It's about offering a hand when the other stumbles and trusting that when the roles reverse, the same hand will be there to steady you.

Our journey hasn't been easy, but it's been ours. And through every trial, we've built an unshakable love that reflects both who we are and who we've become together.

***

Action Steps:

1. **Reflect on Caregiving Roles in Your Relationships**

    Identify a time when you or a loved one has taken on the role of caregiver.

    How did it change your relationship dynamics?

    What lessons did you learn from that experience?

2. **Show Up with Compassion and Understanding**

    Think of one small but meaningful way you can support a partner, friend, or family member today. Whether it's listening, completing a task they find overwhelming, or simply being present, focus on an action that reinforces care and connection.

3. **Prioritize Self-Care**

Recognize that caregiving is a two-way street that requires balance. Reflect on how you can nurture your own emotional and physical well-being.

Commit to one act of self-care this week—something that replenishes your energy and helps you show up for others with strength and kindness.

4. **Foster Open Communication**

Have an honest conversation with someone close to you about the challenges and joys of caregiving.

Share how you can better support one another and set boundaries that honor both of your needs.

5. **Celebrate Small Wins Together**

Acknowledge the victories, no matter how small, in your shared journey. Whether it's overcoming a difficult day or finding a moment of joy, celebrating these milestones strengthens the bond of partnership.

6. **Commitment**
Write down one action you will take this week to show up for a loved one with compassion and one action you'll take to care for yourself.

Reflect on these moments at the end of the week to recognize the strength and resilience that come from balanced caregiving.

***

Closing Reflection

Love, at its core, is about showing up—not just in moments of joy but also in times of uncertainty, vulnerability, and challenge. Our journey as caregivers and partners taught Tony and me that love isn't defined by perfection but by persistence and presence. It's about holding space for each other, embracing the ebbs and flows of life, and finding strength in shared struggles.

As Tony and I navigated the complexities of caregiving and partnership, I learned a profound truth: advocating for love and connection in a relationship mirrors the advocacy we must carry into other aspects of our lives. Whether it's speaking up for a loved one, pushing against societal barriers, or ensuring our own needs are met, advocacy is a constant thread that weaves through every facet of existence.

Our journey as caregivers taught us to trust in each other's strength, even in moments of vulnerability. But it also highlighted the importance of trusting ourselves—our intuition, our experiences, and our voices. Just as I had to advocate for Tony during his recovery, I eventually found myself on a different kind of battlefield, this time fighting for answers in my own health journey.

Self-advocacy can feel isolating and overwhelming, especially in the face of doubt or dismissal. Yet, in these moments, persistence becomes a beacon, guiding us toward clarity and empowerment. My experience with vision loss and the long road to diagnosis revealed that advocating for oneself requires skill and a profound act of self-respect and courage. This understanding reshaped how I approached my care—and how I continue to encourage others to embrace their own journeys.

As we move forward, we'll explore how the power of advocacy transcends relationships and enters the broader realm of healthcare, community, and personal growth. Advocacy begins with a simple but courageous step: believing that your voice is worth being heard.

Full Circle

Lessons and Legacies

Finesse Literary Press Ltd.

11

Advocating for Ourselves

Mini-Lesson: Advocacy is about persistence, patience, and believing in the validity of your own experience.

JUST AS I HAD advocated for Tony during his recovery, I eventually had to advocate for myself—this time as the patient. The journey toward my diagnosis was long, filled with doubt, frustration, and moments of feeling dismissed. Self-advocacy isn't always easy, especially when faced with skepticism or systemic barriers, but it's essential.

Self-advocacy begins with recognizing that your voice matters. However, for many people, self-advocacy can feel daunting, especially within healthcare systems that often fail to see the individual. For me, the journey to a diagnosis was one of persistence, patience, and the unwavering belief in the validity of my lived experience, even when it wasn't immediately validated by others.

The Long Road to Answers

The symptoms began subtly—an inability to see what I knew I should be able to see, a struggle to adjust my eyes to lighting changes, and a nagging sense that something wasn't quite right. Each visit to the optometrist left me more frustrated as the tests consistently showed nothing wrong. My prescribed glasses never fully alleviated the issues.

I repeated the same sentence at every appointment: *"I'm not seeing what I know I'm supposed to see."* Each time, my concerns were dismissed. I began to doubt myself, wondering if I was imagining the problem. The process left me feeling unseen, unheard, and dismissed.

Trusting Myself

In 2013, after years of frustration, I chose to stop driving. The decision wasn't easy. Although it reduced my independence, I knew it was the right thing to do for my safety and that of others. Around this time, during a routine optometrist visit, I impulsively asked for contact lenses. I hoped they might somehow provide clarity that glasses didn't.

When I tried them, my vision became even more distorted. For the first time, the optometrist acknowledged that my issues might warrant further investigation. He referred me to a retinal specialist, a step that would ultimately lead to the answers I had been seeking.

The Power of Persistence

Meeting with the retinal specialist was a turning point. She listened intently as I described my symptoms and tearfully admitted my fears of being dismissed yet again. Her simple but powerful response was, *"I believe you."*

That validation meant everything. It set in motion a series of tests that finally led to my diagnosis of cone rod dystrophy in 2015. Receiving the diagnosis was bittersweet. On one hand, I finally had an explanation for what I was experiencing. On the other, it marked the beginning of a new reality in which I would have to learn to adapt to progressive vision loss.

Lessons in Advocacy

Through this experience, I learned that advocating for yourself in the healthcare system requires resilience and persistence. Here are a few practical lessons I've carried with me:

1. **Trust Your Experience:** No one knows your body better than you do. If something feels wrong, keep seeking answers.

2. **Document Everything:** Keep a record of symptoms, appointments, and test results. This can provide valuable context for healthcare providers.

3. **Find Your Allies:** Seek out professionals who listen and take your concerns seriously. A compassionate provider can make all the difference.

4. **Ask Questions:** Don't hesitate to ask for clarification, second opinions, or alternative approaches. Advocacy starts with understanding your options.

5. **Persist:** If one door closes, find another. Your health and well-being are worth fighting for.

Advocacy as Empowerment

Advocacy is about pushing for what you need and reclaiming your power and agency in the face of uncertainty. This journey taught me to trust my voice, embrace my truth, and take an active role in shaping my care. Getting a diagnosis was the bonus.

I've learned that self-advocacy is essential and transformative. It strengthened my belief in the importance of persistence, the value of connection, and the power of believing in oneself.

***

Action Steps:

Advocating for Ourselves
 1. **Reflect on Your Experiences**
    Think about a time when you felt unheard or

dismissed, whether in a healthcare setting, workplace, or personal relationship.
What were the circumstances, and how did it make you feel?

Did you take steps to advocate for yourself? If so, what worked? If not, what could you have done differently?

2. Identify One Area Where Advocacy Is Needed

Consider a current situation where your needs or concerns are not fully acknowledged.
What outcome are you seeking?

What steps can you take to express your concerns or needs clearly and confidently?

3. Prepare Your Advocacy Tools

Advocacy often requires persistence and organization. Begin building your toolkit:
Write down your concerns and questions to ensure you address them during discussions.

Record key details such as symptoms, dates, and outcomes from past interactions.

Identify allies—whether healthcare providers, colleagues, or friends—who can support and validate your perspective.

4. **Take a Small but Intentional Step**
Commit to one specific action to advocate for yourself this week.

a. Schedule a follow-up appointment, share your concerns with a trusted individual, or research your rights and options.

b. Practice articulating your needs in a way that is clear, confident, and respectful.

5. **Reinforce the Importance of Your Voice**
Advocacy begins with believing that your experiences and needs are valid.
Write down one affirmation that reminds you of your worth: "My voice matters" or "I have the right to be heard."

Keep this affirmation visible as a reminder of your strength and persistence.

6. Celebrate Progress

Advocacy is a journey, not a one-time event. Reflect on your progress, whether it's a small win or a significant breakthrough. Acknowledge the courage it takes to advocate for yourself and use these victories as motivation for future actions.

By taking these steps, you empower yourself to navigate challenges with confidence, persistence, and the knowledge that your voice has the power to create meaningful change.

***

Closing Reflection

Advocating for ourselves can feel like an uphill battle, especially when faced with systemic barriers or skepticism. But in those moments of doubt, remember this: your voice matters, your experiences are valid, and your persistence can pave the way for change. Self-advocacy begins with believing that you are worth fighting for.

Through the long journey of seeking answers, I learned that trusting my voice was as crucial as finding those who believed in it. Advocacy taught me to reclaim my agency and see challenges not as barriers but as opportunities to assert my worth and truth. Persistence is not just a tool—it's a lifeline.

Self-advocacy is often forged in moments of darkness when the path forward seems obscured by pain, uncertainty, or loss. In those moments, it is not persistence but hope that guides us. My self-advocacy journey with vision loss prepared me for greater challenges ahead when darkness seemed to engulf every corner of my life. Yet, even in those shadows, I discovered flickers of light—through community, purpose, and the profound realization that healing often begins with connection.

As we move into the next chapter, let's seek the light that can emerge after darkness. It's not about returning to what once was but about embracing a new and more profound illumination—a light forged by resilience, fueled by community, and filled with possibilities. When life challenges us to redefine ourselves, we find that the light after darkness holds a beauty and strength we may never have known. Let's explore what it means to find hope, healing, and joy beyond the horizon.

12

There is Light After Darkness

Mini-Lesson: The light you find after darkness may be different than before, but it can be even brighter.

DARKNESS HAS A WAY of making time feel suspended, as though each moment stretches endlessly without promise of relief. When I was at my lowest—grieving my diagnosis, living with unrelenting pain, and feeling the weight of uncertainty—I couldn't imagine a way forward. My world had been upended, and I was left to navigate the pieces in unfamiliar terrain. But even in that suffocating darkness, I learned something profound: there is always light, even if it takes time to find it.

That light doesn't always look like what we expect. It doesn't come in grand gestures or instant transformations. For me, it began as the slightest flicker—a kind word, a shared story, and a tiny step toward purpose. Bit by bit, those moments of light became brighter, guiding me toward a new way of seeing the world and myself. They didn't erase the pain or the challenges, but they gave me something far more enduring: hope.

The Darkest Moments

There was a time when my life felt like it had been shattered into pieces. Receiving my diagnosis of cone rod dystrophy was a blow, but it was the persistent daily headache, NDPH, that truly plunged me into darkness. Each day blurred into the next, filled with pain, despair, and a profound sense of loss.

I grieved for the life I'd once had and the future I thought I had lost. Everything felt uncertain. *Would I ever find joy again? Could I rebuild a meaningful life?*

A Flicker of Light

Amid the darkness, a flicker of light appeared—not all at once, but in small, gradual moments. It came in the form of community. Connecting with others who had faced similar struggles reminded me that I was not alone. Their stories of resilience and determination gave me hope that I, too, could find a way forward.

It also came through purpose. Starting my Instagram account, @purposeinview, was a lifeline. What began as a way to document my journey and connect with others became a platform for advocacy, storytelling, and education. Each post was a step toward reclaiming my identity and finding a new sense of self-worth.

Finding Strength in Community

Community has been one of the greatest sources of light in my journey. I found strength in the shared stories, the moments of laughter, and the collective resilience. Whether through social media, advocacy groups, or personal relationships, these connections have been a reminder that we are stronger together.

I've learned that healing doesn't happen in isolation. It's through the support of others—friends, family, and even strangers—that we find the courage to face our challenges and move forward.

Embracing a New Purpose

Adversity can reshape our priorities and reveal strengths we never knew we had. The challenges I faced became the foundation for a new purpose. I realized that my story had the power to inspire, educate, and connect.

Through advocacy, I've had the privilege of breaking barriers, challenging stereotypes, and showing that life with vision loss and chronic illness is not the end—it's a new beginning. I've learned to see beauty in unexpected places and to appreciate the resilience that has carried me through.

Hope Beyond the Horizon

One lesson I've learned through this journey is that hope is always within reach. Even when the path is unclear and the light seems distant, it is there—waiting for us to take the next step.

Finding light after darkness means uncovering hope in unexpected places, creating purpose from adversity, and recognizing that beauty and strength can emerge from the cracks even when life feels broken.

The light I discovered after darkness is more nuanced than before, shaped by the challenges I've faced and the lessons I've learned. It is also brighter because it is filled with the richness of resilience, the depth of community, and the boundless possibilities of purpose.

***

Action Steps:

1. **Reflect on Your Journey**
   Recall a time in your life when you faced a period of darkness or challenge. Write down the small moments or actions that began to bring light into your life, such as a meaningful conversation, a personal accomplishment, or a connection with someone who understood your struggles.

2. **Identify One Step Forward**
   Think of one tangible step you can take today to create or seek light in your life. This could be

as simple as reaching out to a supportive friend, journaling about your feelings, pursuing a creative outlet, or exploring a new community that aligns with your values and experiences.

3. **Celebrate Small Wins**

Commit to noticing and celebrating even the smallest moments of progress or positivity in your life. Whether it's a shared laugh, a new perspective, or an act of kindness, acknowledging these moments reinforces hope and resilience.

4. **Build Connections**

Consider how you can connect with others who may share similar challenges or journeys. Joining a support group, participating in an online forum, or simply sharing your story can foster mutual encouragement and light for yourself and others.

5. **Embrace Purpose**

Reflect on how your experiences might guide you toward a greater sense of purpose. Think about how you can use what you've learned to inspire or support others. Write down one way you can channel your story into something meaningful, such as advocacy, mentoring, or creative expression.

By engaging in these actions, you can take intentional steps toward rediscovering hope, embracing resilience, and creating a brighter path forward.

***

Closing Reflection

The journey from darkness to light isn't about erasing the pain or forgetting the struggles; it's about transforming them into something meaningful. The cracks that once threatened to break us become spaces where light enters, illuminating the strength and beauty we carry within.

The light we find after darkness is different from what we knew before. It is shaped by the resilience we've built, the connections we've made, and the lessons we've learned. It is a light of clarity, purpose, and a deeper understanding of what truly matters.

As I reflect on my journey, I know that darkness is not the end of the story—it's a chapter. And like all chapters, it leads to something new. The light holds the promise of not just surviving but thriving and not just moving forward but creating a life filled with meaning, connection, and joy.

To anyone navigating their own darkness: hold on. The light may seem distant, but it is there. It may not look like what you expect, but it will guide you to a version of yourself that is stronger, wiser, and more whole. Even after the darkest nights, dawn always comes. And when it does, it brings a light that can be even more beautiful than you ever imagined.

13

A Call to Action

Mini-Lesson: Each of us has the power to create change, whether in our own lives or the world around us.

As the light after darkness reveals new possibilities, it invites us to take the next step—to embrace our growth and extend that light outward. Advocacy and inclusivity are not solitary endeavors; they are movements fueled by collective action and shared purpose. The challenges we overcome equip us with unique insights and the power to create meaningful change. Now is the time to harness that power, turn lessons into action, and answer the call to shape a world where everyone, regardless of their abilities, feels seen, valued, and empowered.

Change often feels overwhelming, as though it requires grand gestures or boundless resources. But the truth is, change begins with each of us—one choice, one action, and one moment at a time. The work of creating a more inclusive and connected world is not reserved for a select few; it's a shared responsibility.

Empowerment Through Action

Advocacy starts with the belief that our experiences matter. Self-advocacy helped me navigate my challenges, but it also revealed a greater truth: the ripple effect of standing up for yourself inspires others to do the same.

Whether it's speaking out against injustices, educating others about accessibility, or making intentional choices to include and uplift marginalized voices, every action matters. Change doesn't happen overnight but builds with every small step forward.

Building a Movement

No movement for inclusivity happens in isolation; it thrives in community. The power of collective voices amplifies the impact of individual efforts. Over the years, I've been privileged to witness the transformative power of community. Together, we've challenged stereotypes, expanded access, and shifted perceptions about what's possible.

But there is still so much work to be done. True inclusivity requires all of us to examine our biases, rethink our assumptions, and commit to doing better— for ourselves and for the generations to come.

Small Steps, Big Impact

Change doesn't have to be monumental to be meaningful. Here are some simple actions you can take to make a difference:

1. **Educate Yourself:** Learn about the experiences of people with disabilities. Follow advocates and organizations that are creating accessible spaces.

2. **Practice Accessibility:** When creating content, hosting events, or engaging online, think about how to make it accessible for everyone. Use tools

like alt text, captions, and accessible design.

3. **Support Local Advocates:** Amplify the voices of those already doing the work. Share their content, attend their events, and engage with their stories.

4. **Have Conversations:** Talk to friends, family, and colleagues about inclusivity. Ask questions, share insights, and challenge stereotypes.

5. **Advocate for Change:** Speak up when you see barriers to inclusion—at work, in your community, or online.

An Invitation to Join

The journey toward inclusivity and advocacy is ongoing, and each of us needs to play a part. Whether you're just starting out or have been advocating for years, your voice and actions are vital.

Together, we can create a world where differences are celebrated, where accessibility is the norm, and where no one feels left behind.

***

Action Steps:

Advocate for Inclusivity

1. **Identify an Area for Change**

    Reflect on one specific area in your life or community where inclusivity could be improved. This could be at work, in a social setting, or online. Ask yourself:

    Where do I see barriers, and how can I help remove them?

2. **Set a Concrete Goal**

    Decide on one tangible step you can take to address this area. Examples include:

    a. Adding alt text and captions to your social media posts.

    b. Suggesting accessibility improvements at your workplace or community events.

c. Starting a conversation with a friend or colleague about inclusivity.

3. Educate Yourself

Spend time learning about the experiences and needs of people with disabilities or marginalized voices. Follow advocates, read articles, or take courses to deepen your understanding of accessibility.

4. Engage in Advocacy

Take one intentional action this week:

a. Write an email proposing changes that enhance accessibility.

b. Share content from an advocate or organization that resonates with you.

c. Practice using inclusive language in your conversations.

5. Reflect on Your Impact

After taking action, consider its impact. Did it spark a conversation, create awareness, orinspire change? Use this reflection to plan your next step toward advocacy.

Remember, every small action matters. By starting today, you become part of a larger movement for inclusivity and positive change.

***

Closing Reflection

Change doesn't begin with others; it begins with us. Each of us has the power to create ripples of impact that extend far beyond what we can see. By embracing our roles as advocates, allies, and changemakers, we can build a future where everyone belongs.

Let's commit to being the spark for the change we wish to see. Together, we can illuminate a path toward a world that is more inclusive, more compassionate, and more connected. The call to action is clear. The time to act is now.

Conclusion

I'll never forget the message I received from that young girl years ago. Seeing someone who looked like her using a white cane gave her the courage to embrace her identity with confidence. For the first time, she felt seen, not just as someone navigating vision loss but as someone with a story that mattered. Her words carried a weight that shifted my entire perception of myself and toward vision loss. I realized then that our stories are not just for ourselves—they ripple outward, touching lives in ways we might never fully see. That simple, powerful connection reminded me that even in darkness, light can be found through shared humanity.

This book has been a reflection of my journey and the lessons I've learned through grief, resilience, and transformation. At its core, the message is clear: life's challenges, no matter how overwhelming, hold within them the potential for growth, connection, and purpose. Advocacy, representation, and storytelling are bridges to understanding and inclusion, helping us build a world where no one feels left behind.

Lessons From the Journey

As I reflect on each chapter, I see the roadmap that has guided me:

- **Owning Our Stories** taught me that it takes courage to embrace vulnerability and rewrite the narratives that have held us back.

- **Finding Our Voice** was a reminder that speaking up is not just for ourselves—it's a way to inspire and empower others.

- **Building Resilience** showed me the strength that emerges from adversity and the importance of equipping ourselves with the tools to persevere.

- **Representation Matters** underscored the profound impact of seeing ourselves reflected in spaces where we've historically been excluded.

- **Becoming Advocates** demonstrated the power of persistence, patience, and believing in the validity of our experiences.

- **Community and Connection** reaffirmed that healing and growth thrive in the presence of support, shared stories, and mutual understanding.

- **Purpose After Pain** revealed how even the most difficult experiences can lead us to deeper meaning and fulfillment.

- **There Is Light After Darkness** reminded me that while the light we find may be different than before, it often shines even brighter, shaped by resilience, hope, and a newfound clarity of purpose.

Each chapter is a step on the path toward living authentically, advocating boldly, and creating a more inclusive and compassionate world.

A Call to Action

As you close this book, take a moment to reflect on your own story. What challenges have shaped you? What moments of light have guided you through darkness? How can you use your voice, your experiences, and your unique perspective to make an impact?

You don't need to have it all figured out to take the first step. Start small. Advocate for yourself or someone else. Share your story, even if your voice shakes. Seek out connection and community. And above all, believe in the power of your journey.

Your voice matters. Your experiences are valid. Your story is worth sharing. Each step you take, no matter how small, has the potential to inspire others, spark change, and illuminate the way forward.

A Message of Hope

This journey has taught me that the darkness we face does not define us. How we navigate that darkness—how we seek out light, hold onto hope, and lean into connection—reveals our true strength.

The light after darkness is not simply a return to what was; it is a transformation. It is a new way of seeing, shaped by resilience, community, and a profound sense of purpose. And often, it is even more beautiful than we could have imagined.

RESILIENCE AND PURPOSE

Together, we can build a world where everyone feels seen, valued, and empowered to thrive. There is always light after darkness. And that light begins with you.

Acknowledgements

No book is written alone, and this one is no exception. It has been shaped, supported, and strengthened by the incredible people who have walked alongside me on this journey.

To my husband, Tony—your love, patience, and unwavering support have been my foundation. You have seen me at my strongest and my most vulnerable, and through it all, you have stood by my side, believing in me even when I struggled to believe in myself. I am forever grateful for your love and partnership.

To my children, Chenessa, Christopher, and Lauren—you are my greatest teachers. Watching you grow has shown me the power of resilience, the beauty of unconditional love, and the importance of leaving a legacy that matters. I hope this book reminds you that even in life's hardest moments, there is always light waiting to be found. You are the authors of your own stories—may you write them boldly, fearlessly, and with hearts full of purpose.

To my publisher and the entire Finesse Literary Press team—thank you for believing in this story and for working tirelessly to bring it to life. Your dedication and support to me means more than I can express.

To my fellow advocates, friends, and mentors who have inspired me and reminded me that our voices matter—thank you for your wisdom, encouragement, and the work you do to make this world a more inclusive place.

To my community—whether you are a reader, a listener, a supporter on social media, or someone walking a similar journey—thank you. Your stories, messages, and shared experiences have reinforced why this work matters. This book is for all of us who have faced adversity and chosen to turn it into strength.

And lastly, to my past self—the girl who was afraid of what the future might hold—thank you for holding on, for finding light in the cracks, and for choosing to move forward even when the path wasn't clear.

With gratitude,
Anne Mok

Endnotes

1. Mok, Anne. *@purposeinview*. Instagram, 2020.

2. Aille Design. *Aille: pronounced eye*, 2025, ailledesign.com.

3. Purdys Chocolatiers. *Assorted Chocolate Braille Gift Box*, 2025, purdys.com.

4. Specsavers. 2025, specsavers.ca.

5. United Nations Convention on the Rights of Persons with Disabilities (2006). From the Preamble (e) to the CRPD. https:\\www.ohchr.org/en/hrbodies/crpd/pages/conventionrightspersonswithdisabilities.aspx

6. Kvenberg, Sabine. *Become Empowered: Echoes of Grace and Strength*. Impact Publishers, 2024.

7. McCoy, Stephanae. *Bold Blind Beauty*, 2025, boldblindbeauty.com.

8. Harris, Jillian. *The Jilly Academy*, 2021, jillyacademy.jillianharris.com.

9. Harris, Jillian. *A Candid Conversation with Alumni Member Anne on Finding Purpose in Entrepreneurship*, May 2022, jillianharris.com.

With Readience & Respect.
Lola.
Anne

With Resilience & Purpose,
 Love,
  Anne